'WHEN YOU'RE
AROUND ME,
YOU'RE GOING
TO GET GLITTER
ON YOU.'

Kesha

CONTENTS

YOUR ULTIMATE GLITTER PLAYLIST

AFTER THE GLITTER FADES – Stevie Nicks

SPARKLE – Diana Ross

GLITTER IN THE AIR – Pink

SPARKLE – No Doubt

PUT ME IN A MOVIE – Lana Del Rey

RAZZLE DAZZLE – Chicago

DIAMONDS ARE A GIRL'S BEST FRIEND – Marilyn Monroe

DIAMONDS – Rihanna

WILDSTAR – Giorgio Moroder (feat. Foxes)

GOLD – Prince

EVERYTHING THAT GLITTERS – Pusha T (feat. French Montana)

GLITTER YEARS – The Bangles

BAUBLES, BANGLES AND BEADS – Nina Simone

CONFETTI – Sia

A KIND OF MAGIC – Queen

FANTASY – Maria Carey

GLAMOUR GIRL – Chicks on Speed

RUBY – Kaiser Chiefs

24K MAGIC – Bruno Mars

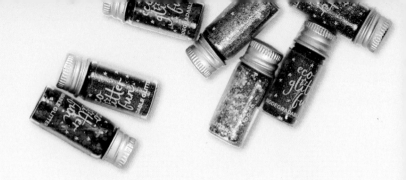

GLAM UP THE GOOD TIMES

In a world where voices are getting louder, protests noticed and individuality embraced, there's one kaleidoscopic entity that mirrors the energy of those standing up, ready to be heard. Glitter offers a wash-away, one-night-only transformation that enables us to become somebody, and even something else, transcending the everyday.

Glitter means good times and even better vibes. It's a simple sign that you're ready to turn heads and let others take notice. And have fun doing it all. Whether it's elevating your festival get-up with bejewelled face adornments, a loud-and-proud glitter beard on a Saturday night out, or a pair of shoes so sparkly that Dorothy's ruby slippers simply fade into the background, there are millions of ways to embrace a little glitter in your life.

From the different ways to shimmer and shine, to expert top tips and how to wash it all away in an environmentally responsible way, your one-stop guide to glitter starts here.

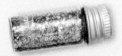

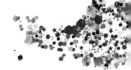

GLITTER KIT

Please Glitter Responsibly

Like most good things we love, there is a downside to wearing glitter. While on the surface it sparkles with splendour, when washed down the drain it can have a serious, harmful effect on the environment.

Before you choose your glitter shade and style, consider its provenance and the effect it will have once you've washed it away. It's chic to shine, but chicer to shine responsibly.

Our 7 Favourite Eco-Friendly Glitter Brands

Eco Stardust:
ecostardust.com

The Mermaid Cave:
the-mermaid-cave.co.uk

Eco Glitter Fun:
ecoglitterfun.com

Festival Face:
festivalface.co.uk

Bio Glitz:
bioglitz.co

Projekt:
projektglitter.com

Bleach London:
bleachlondon.co.uk

Glue/Fixing Sprays:
Glitter Fix: gogetglitter.com
Urban Decay All Nighter
Setting Spray: urbandecay.co.uk
Elnette hairspray: boots.com

Brushes:
spectrumcollections.com

Eyeshadow:
maccosmetics.co.uk

Gems:
thegypsyshrine.com

Sequins:
hobbycraft.co.uk

Body Tape:
Boots Microporous
Surgical Tape: boots.com

HOW TO REMOVE GLITTER

If you thought applying glitter was messy, just wait until the time comes to take it all off. Glitter gets everywhere. It's unavoidable and part of the fun.

Start in a place where you don't have to worry about letting speckles fly.

How to Remove Eye Make-Up

You're going to need a steady hand to direct make-up off the face and not into your eyes. Don't rub! Dab, hold and swipe – and always go back with a clean surface. Choose an oil-based product that will lift excess quicker.

- Douse a cotton pad with eye make-up remover and, with your eye closed, place the pad over the glitter area.

- Slowly but firmly press down on the pad and glide away from the nose. Repeat until the majority of the glitter has gone.

- Splash face with water and lather with cleanser to remove excess glitter.

- Wipe away gently with a muslin cloth.

- Finish by moisturising skin.

How to Remove Glitter Nail Varnish

Sit back and relish a moment when you can't do anything else. Quite literally.

- Apply a liberal amount of nail-varnish remover to a piece of cotton wool large enough to cover the whole nail.

- Cut a strip of kitchen foil and use it to strap the cotton wool to the nail.

- By the time you've covered all fingers (about ten minutes), the glitter will have broken down. After removing the foil, use gentle force to wipe away the glitter with the cotton wool.

- Use a clean pad to remove any excess.

- To ensure nails remain strong, buff the surface and then treat the cuticle with nourishing oil.

How to Remove Hair Glitter

The longer the hair, the trickier it will be to ensure that every last morsel of glitter is well and truly gone. Perhaps get someone to help; otherwise, patience is key. You might find that you don't want to use your best shampoo immediately, but once the glitter is gone, shampoo and condition as usual.

o If you have gems and rhinestones in your hair, remove these first. Then, using a brush that you don't mind getting glittered, brush through the lengths of your hair.

✕ Wet hair and quickly lather with a sizeable amount of shampoo. Those with thick or textured hair might find it easier to do this in sections.

• Repeat until the water runs clear, and follow up with your usual hair-care routine.

TOP TIP:
Those who are willing to go the extra mile will find that adding coconut oil before the first wash will make for a neater execution and nourishing finish.

How to Remove Body Glitter

Don't think you're going to need to trade in your bubble bath for a mass of eye make-up remover to take off your snazzy shoulder shimmer. The force of a shower met with a good amount of body wash will work just fine. A loofah will help, but don't scrub or scrape.

o Step into the shower and gently wipe away the glitter.

-¦- Lather the body wash into the loofah or flannel and wipe away any of the more stubborn pieces that remain.

o Once out of the shower and dried off, use moisturiser to restore and repair skin.

1

SEE THE RAINBOW

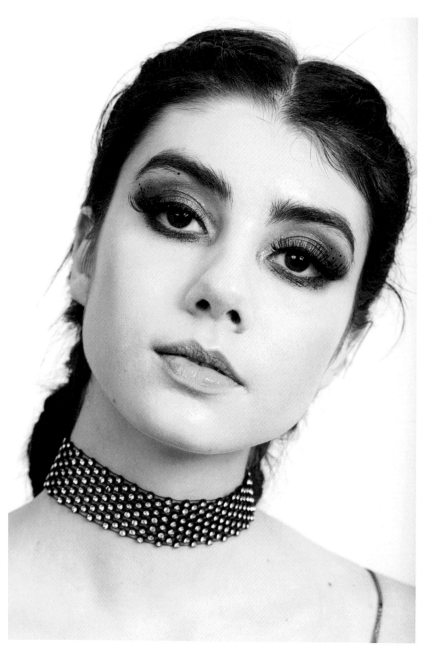

1
SEE THE RAINBOW

This might be a step-by-step to a perfect gradient of colour-chart heaven, but don't think that this is the only way to do it. Mix shades, go stripy, or do three parts one colour to two parts a contrasting colour. You'll soon be the Matisse of make-up.

What you need:

Primer

White eyeliner

Eyeshadow in at least three contrasting shades, including white

Cosmetic glitter in at least three contrasting shades

Make-up glue

Fixing spray

Mascara

Eye brushes for each colour and each glitter shade

o Apply primer to the eyelid.

-¦- Once set, mark out the colours with the white eyeliner across the eyelid. Mark larger sections in the centre and smaller sections towards the outer edges.

o Apply the eyeshadow colour by colour, before blending for a seamless finish.

. Apply the glue on top of the first colour and swiftly add the coordinating glitter on top. Make sure that the glitters blend by repeating, if necessary.

✕ Finish with a spritz of fixing spray and a few layers of mascara.

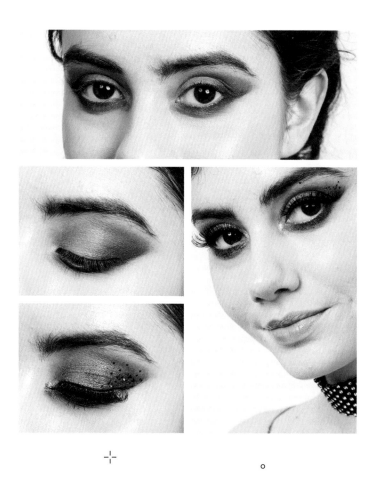

'MY FAVOURITE COLOUR IS SHINY.'
Marc Jacobs

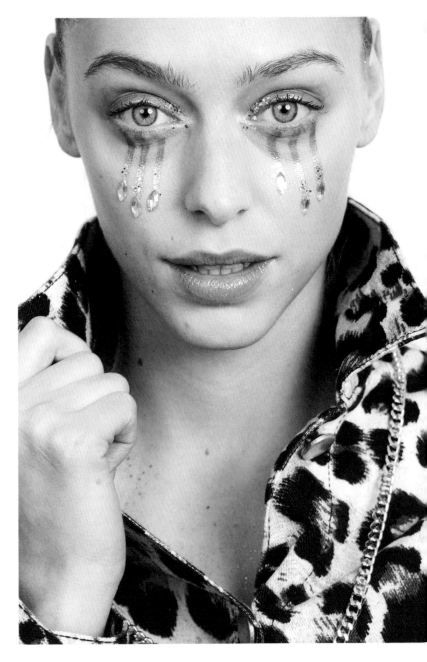

2

CRY ME A GLITTER TEAR

2
CRY ME A GLITTER TEAR

There's nothing sad going on here. This look has potential for all manner of occasions. Reshuffle shades and combinations for a spooky doll at Halloween, a mythical fairy at Glastonbury, or just an all-out glitter ball come New Year's Eve.

What you need:

Eyeshadow

Eyeliner

Make-up glue

Cosmetic glitter

Gems (optional)

- o Once you've applied your eyeshadow to the lid, it's time to get creative.

- ⊣⊢ From the lash line to your cheekbone, mark out three lines of differing lengths with the eyeliner.

- o With the eyeshadow, lightly dust over the eyeliner markings to create wider 'tears'.

- . Apply the glue over the eyeshadow and dab on the glitter, applying it more densely at the bottom.

- ✕ Why not finish with a gem at the bottom for a nice touch?

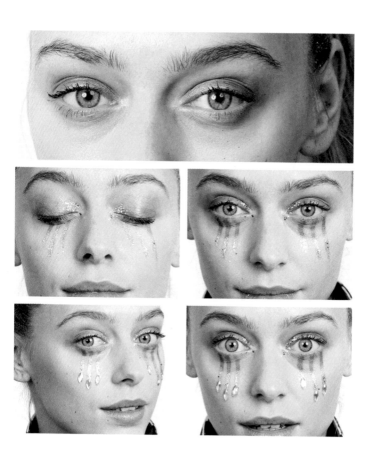

3
GLITTER WATERLINE

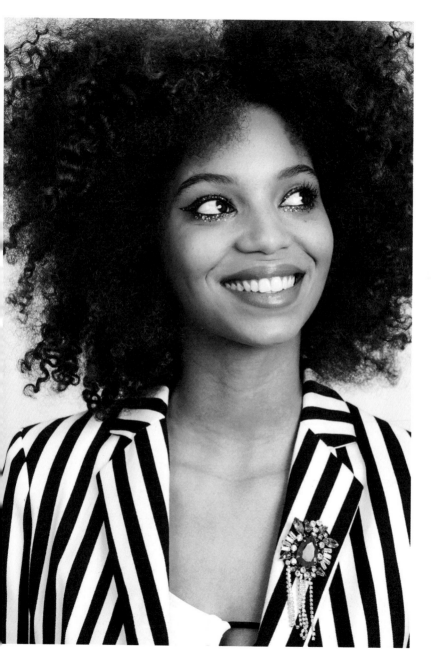

3
GLITTER WATERLINE

Think of this one as the eyeshadow version of a mullet: business as usual up top, and a party down below. Stick to your usual go-to for the lid, and let your creativity run wild along the waterline. Those with a steady hand and a penchant for technicolour should trial a rainbow style for ultimate impact.

What you need:

Eyeliner pencil

Liquid glitter eyeliner

Mascara in colour of your choice

o Colour along the waterline and lower lash line with the eyeliner pencil. Extend below more than you usually would for bolder results.

-¦- Focusing below the lower eyelashes only, apply the glitter eyeliner on top of the eyeliner pencil.

o Allow it to dry and repeat until you get the perfect glitter coverage.

. Finish with several coats of mascara on the lower lash line.

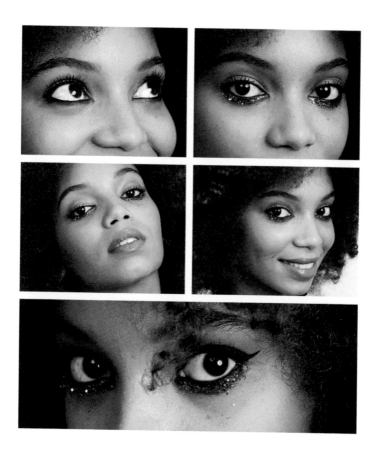

19

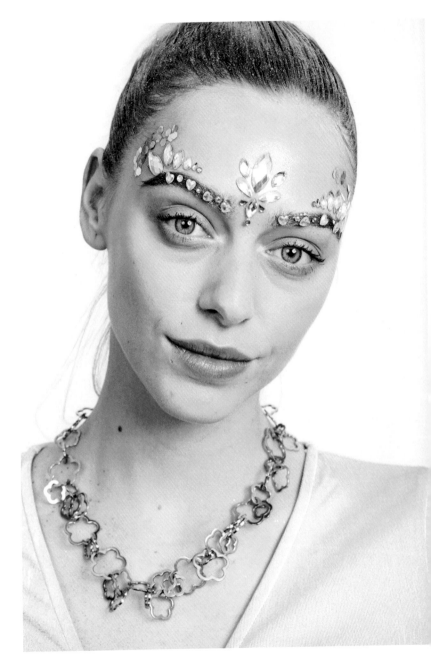

4

GLITTER BEADED BROW

4
GLITTER BEADED BROW

Glitter eyebrows not enough
for your glitter addiction?
This might be just the answer.
A festival classic that we think
has the sass to go the distance.

What you need:

Eyeshadow in two differing shades

Make-up glue

Cosmetic glitter

Gems

Eyeshadow brush

o   Start by filling in your
    eyebrows with the lighter
    shade of eyeshadow.

-¦- Once covered, blend in the
    darker colour, moving from
    the outer edges to the centre.

o   Apply the glue and then
    gently, using fingertips,
    dab on the glitter.

.   Once set, add more glue
    to the exact locations you
    want to place the gems and
    then carefully add them on.

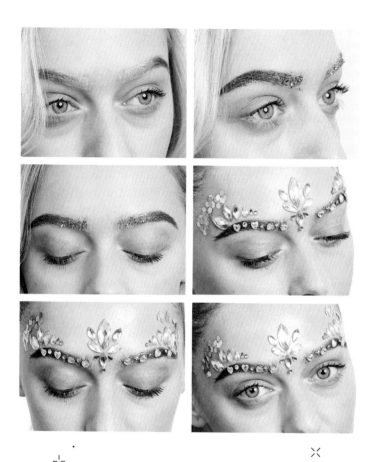

'IF GOD WANTED US TO BEND OVER
HE'D PUT DIAMONDS ON THE FLOOR.'

Joan Rivers

5
THE MASK OF MIRRORS

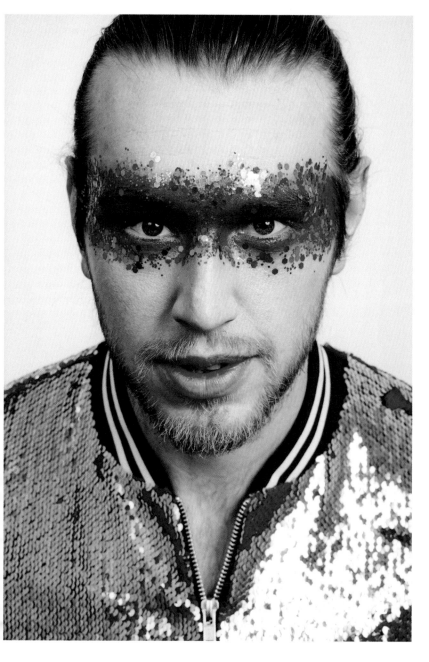

5
THE MASK OF MIRRORS

There's no need to hide with this one. It's a high-impact look, perfect to have in your catalogue for all manner of glitter-is-necessary events – whether it's a masquerade ball or superhero fancy dress.

What you need:

Eyeliner

Metallic eyeshadow

Cosmetic glitter

Sequins

Fixing spray

Eyeshadow brush

o Ensuring that the skin is clean, mark out a mask-like shape around your eye area with eyeliner (above or below the eyebrow, as preferred).

✕ Next, fill the shape in densely with the eyeshadow.

. Take a brush and gently dust the glitter around the far edges, extending from the middle of your eyebrows to the middle of the lower lashes.

o Spritz with fixing spray.

✕ Squirt a scant amount of the glue on the back of a selection of sequins of varying size and place them close – but not too close – to the outer corners of the eye and all around the edges of the mask.

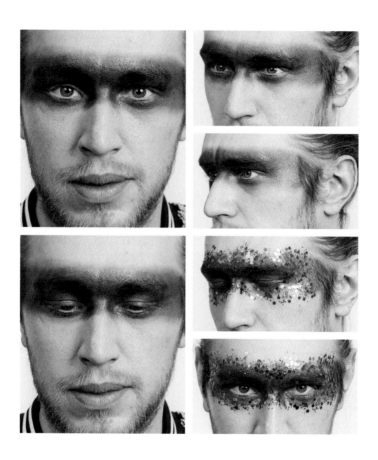

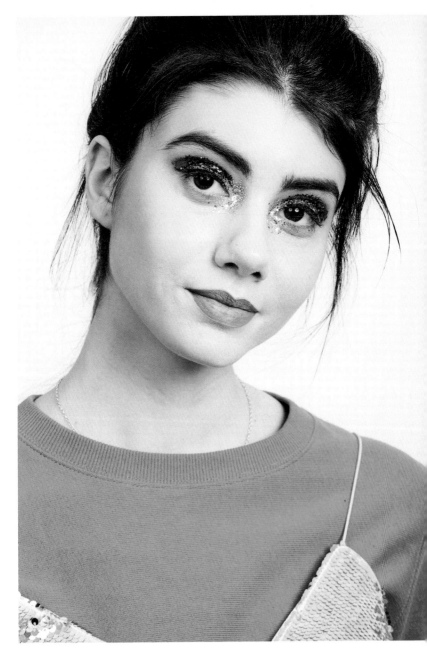

6

GLITTER INNER EYE

6
GLITTER INNER EYE

This is the cut crease (see page 40) turned up full volume. It follows the same steps but ups the ante on the shine front. If the cut crease is about delicate precision, this look is about pure party realness.

What you need:

Primer

Two eyeshadows in a pale and darker shade

Make-up glue

Cosmetic glitter in two shades

Fixing spray

Mascara

o Apply primer to the lid.

✕ Take the lightest eyeshadow and apply it all over the lid, then follow up with the darker shade, extending it up to your eye's crease.

. Apply the glue over the darker shadow and, before it sets, gently apply the glitter.

o Next, using fingertips, carefully apply the second shade of sparkle in the corner of the eyes.

-¦- Finish with a spritz of fixing spray and a few layers of mascara.

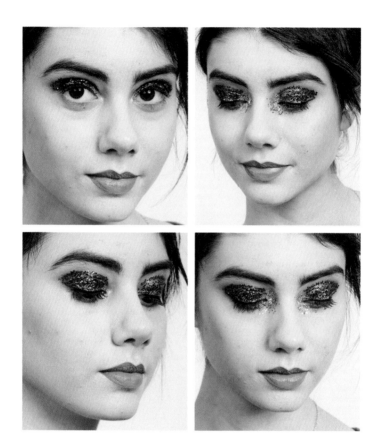

'I QUITE LOVE SEQUINS; I THINK
IT'S THE DRAG QUEEN IN ME.'

Sienna Miller

7

BLINGING BROWS

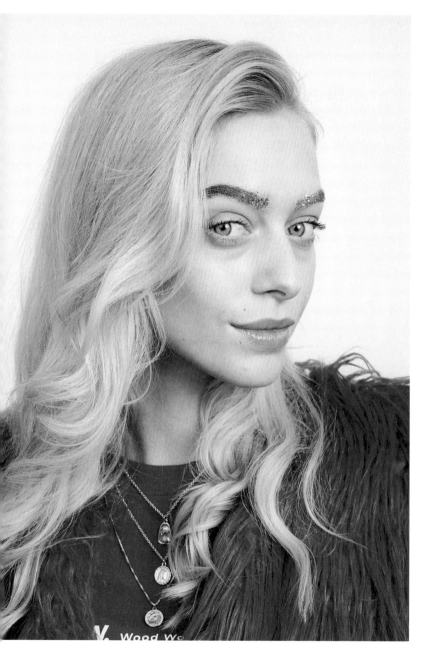

7
BLINGING BROWS

If the eyes are the window to the soul, then that makes brows the curtains. No one wants to be greeted with a boring set, so get ready to make them sparkle. This is a great place to start when getting to grips with glitter beauty, and takes no longer than five minutes.

What you need:

Eyeshadow (optional)

Make-up glue

Cosmetic glitter

Make-up remover (optional)

Cotton bud (optional)

Fixing spray

Two clean eyeshadow brushes

o Starting with clean brows, apply the eyeshadow – if using – in small strokes in the same direction as hair growth, until the brow is fully filled in.

✕ Apply the make-up glue over the brow to set the eyeshadow and hairs in place.

. Working quickly, start close to the nose and dust the glitter across the brows with the second brush. Depending on the desired effect, be as liberal as you wish.

. If you want an immaculate look, clear away any residue or glitter that has fallen out of place with make-up remover and a cotton bud.

-¦- Close eyes and spritz brows with fixing spray.

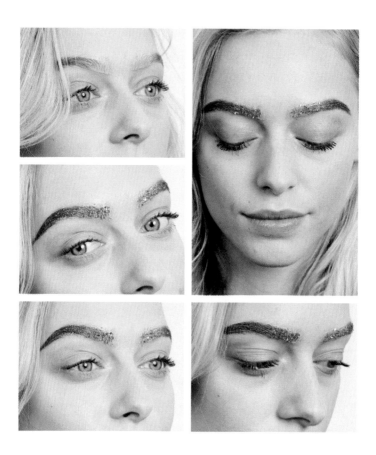

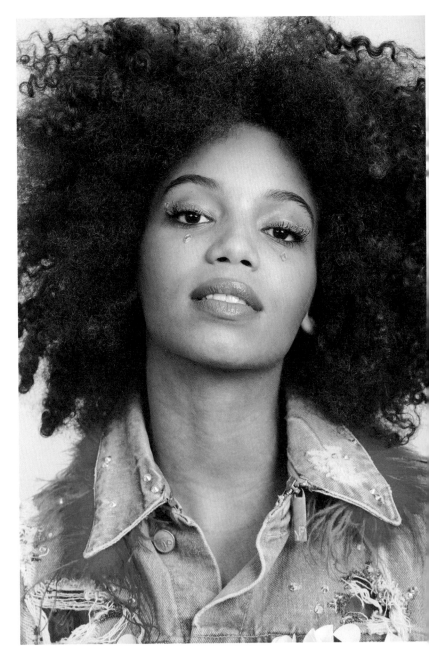

FLUTTER FABULOUS
EYELASHES

8
FLUTTER-FABULOUS EYELASHES

Who doesn't love mascara? So, imagine how much you'll love this look when glitter gets introduced. Colour can really change the way this one works out; don't underestimate the power of a subtle silver over natural-coloured lashes. Chic. Pre-glittered eyelashes are more readily available, but where's the fun in that?

What you need

False eyelashes

Nail varnish in a colour of your choice (optional)

Eyelash glue

Cosmetic glitter sprinkled on a clean plate

Mascara

Tweezers

Small paintbrush

o Comb through the false eyelashes and place on a clean, protected surface.

✕ While holding the lashes with tweezers, gently paint the lashes from root to tip with nail varnish, if using.

. Comb through the lashes before the varnish dries.

o Once dry, take the paintbrush and apply the lash glue to the lashes. Cover just the middle tips or, for a bolder look, cover the whole lashes.

o While the glue is still wet, use tweezers to dip each lash in the glitter laid out on the plate, ensuring that it is evenly distributed across the lashes. Shake any excess glitter away and repeat if necessary.

-¦- Once the glitter is fully dry, apply the lashes as per the packet instructions to complete your beauty look.

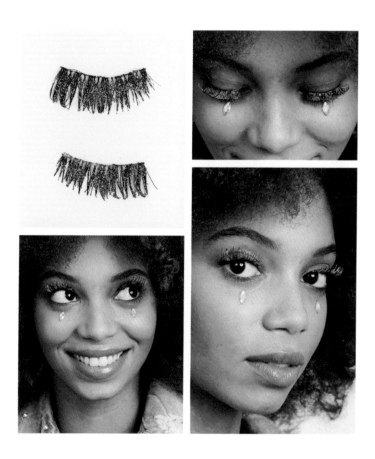

9

THE GO-ALL-OUT GLITTER CUT-CREASE

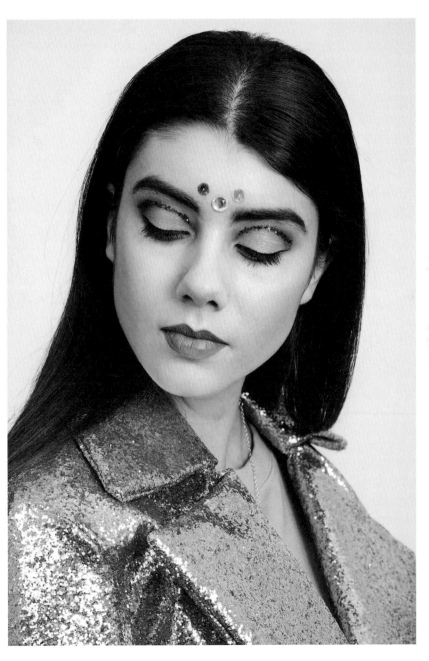

9
THE GO-ALL-OUT GLITTER CUT-CREASE

Many a beauty obsessive will have spent hours in front of the mirror perfecting a cut-crease, where the crease of the eye acts as a natural guide. Adding glitter into the mix will further impress others with a well-trained eye. We're into one gradual shade when it comes to this look.

What you need:

Primer	Black liquid eyeliner
Coordinating eyeliner	Fixing spray
Two eyeshadows in a lighter and darker shade	Mascara
Make-up glue	
Cosmetic glitter	

o Apply primer to the lid.

✕ Once set, mark out the cut crease with the coloured eyeliner just above your natural crease.

. Apply the lightest eyeshadow all over the lid and then follow up with the darker shade over the marked-out cut crease.

o Next, create a cat-eye effect with the black liquid eyeliner.

┴ Over the coloured eyeliner, apply the make-up glue and then carefully add the glitter on top.

. Finish with a spritz of fixing spray and a few layers of mascara.

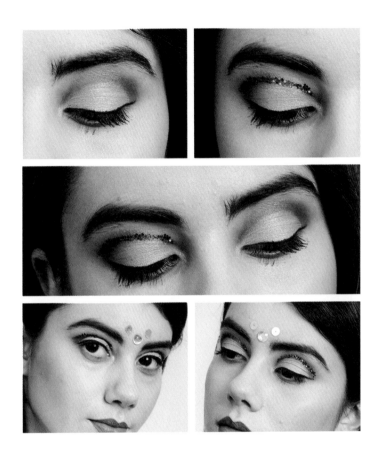

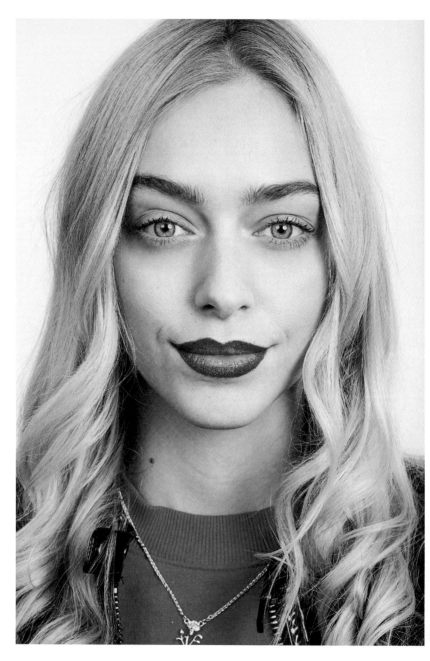

10

THE SUNRISE SMOOCH

10
THE SUNRISE SMOOCH

Sometimes less is more, and while this isn't territory that glitter often finds itself in, it's worth considering going back to basics. Whether you're not looking for the megawatt impact glitter lips offer, or you've mastered that and are looking for a new challenge, these sunrise lips should not be left out of your look book. A nude base is our current daytime favourite.

What you need:

Lip liner

Matte liquid lipstick

Make-up glue

Cosmetic glitter in a contrasting colour

Fixing spray

Two lip brushes

o Mark the shape of the lips with the lip liner and fill them in completely.

✂ Over the liner, apply the liquid lipstick and blot before adding a second coat.

• Apply glue to the centre of the lips and, working outwards, before it dries, liberally apply the glitter at the centre and graduate outwards. You can then brush away any excess product once it is fully coated.

o Spritz lips with fixing spray.

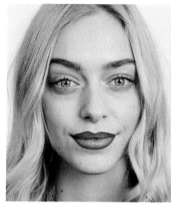

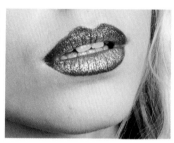

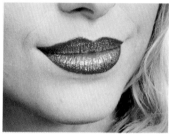

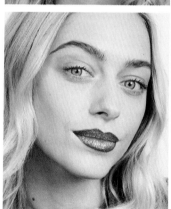

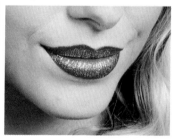

'SOME GIRLS ARE JUST BORN
WITH GLITTER IN THEIR VEINS.'

Paris Hilton

GIVE A GLITTER KISS

11
GIVE A GLITTER KISS

The original and arguably the best. The glitter trend started here, and this effective, easy and surprisingly wearable sparkle will change the way you think of a statement lip forever. It's no surprise that Taylor Swift, Bella Hadid and Rihanna have rocked this look. The trick? It's all in the base.

What you need:

Lip liner

Matte liquid lipstick

Make-up glue

Cosmetic glitter

Fixing spray

Two lip brushes

o Mark the shape of the lips with the liner and fill them in completely.

✕ Over the liner, apply the liquid lipstick and blot before adding a second coat.

. Apply a layer of glue to the lips and, before it dries, liberally apply the glitter. You can then brush away any excess product once it is fully coated.

o Spritz lips with fixing spray.

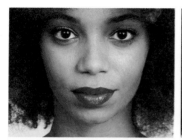
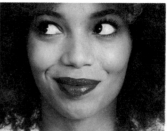
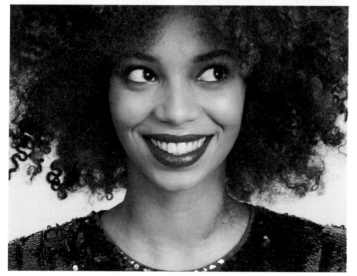

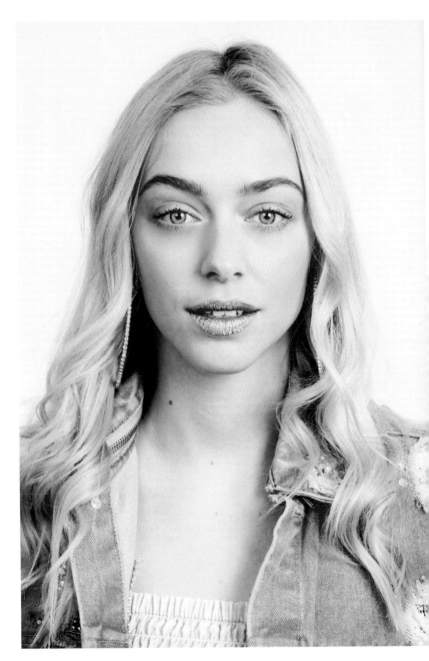

12

THE SHINING LINE

12
THE SHINING LINE

Kylie Jenner has a lot to answer for. The beauty mogul has more or less single-handedly brought back lip liner. For this look, forget the everyday go-to nudes you love and embrace the flamboyant. Sticking to one colour works well, but strike out with a contrast palette if you dare.

What you need:

Lip liner in nude and a contrast colour (optional)

Matte liquid lipstick

Make-up glue

A contrast colour cosmetic glitter

Fixing spray

Three lip brushes

o   Mark the shape of the lips with the liner and fill them in completely.

✕   Over the liner, apply the liquid lipstick and blot before adding a second coat.

·   If using a contrast colour, apply that now. If not, place the glue around the edge of the lips and apply your chosen glitter. Brush away any residue with a clean brush.

o   Spritz lips with fixing spray.

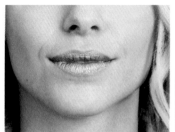
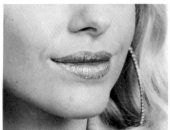
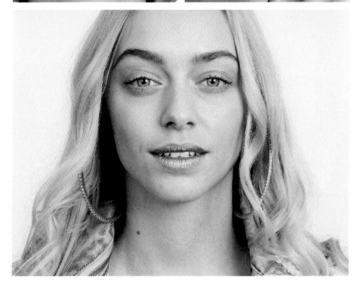

13

RHINESTONE LIPS

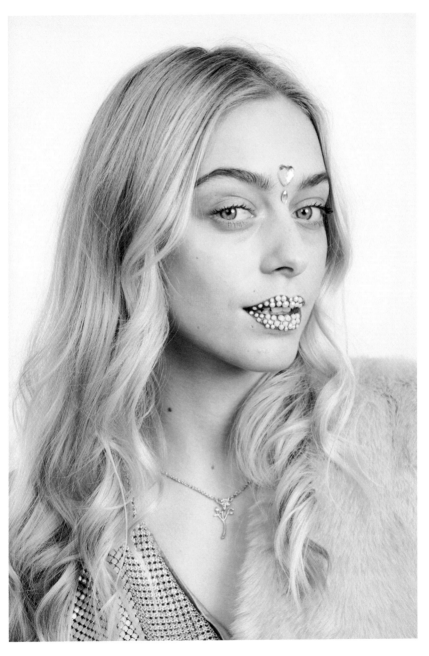

13
RHINESTONE LIPS

Turn the impact volume up. This rhinestone lip look is for scene-stealers and dancing queens. The ultimate selfie accessory that feels right out of the catalogue of the disco-fever seventies. You will need patience here, but – trust us – it's worth it.

What you need:

Lip liner

Matte liquid lipstick

Make-up glue

Rhinestones

Fixing spray

Tweezers

o   Mark the shape of the lips with the liner and fill them in completely.

⋊⋉   Over the liner, apply the liquid lipstick and blot before adding a second coat.

.   Add the glue to the back of a rhinestone and attach it to the centre of the lip. Repeat for each one, applying them from the centre of the lip outwards.

o   Spritz lips with fixing spray.

TOP TIP:
Go bold – choose different shapes and colours for pic'n'mix panache.

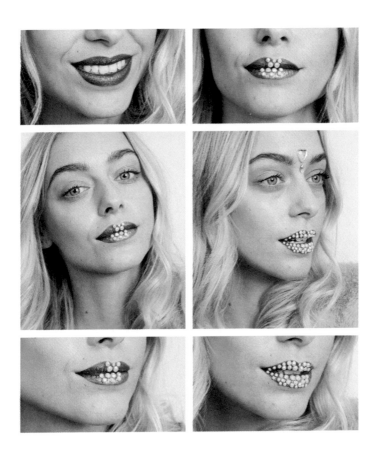

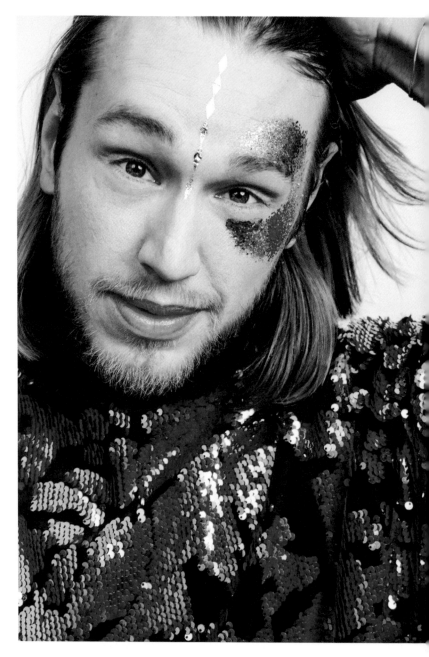

14

CONTOUR 2.0

14
CONTOUR 2.0

Define those killer cheekbones or your favourite facial features all the more by strobing with sparkle. Keep it neutral to your skin tone for a subtler touch, or be extravagant with standout colours that strike a different chord.

What you need:

Eyeshadow (optional)

Make-up glue

Cosmetic glitter in multiple shades

Fixing spray

Contour brush

o   If using eyeshadow, shade the areas of the face that you want to contour.

✕   Buff the shade in so that it blends easily.

.   Apply make-up glue over the eyeshadow, then gently add the glitter on top, shade by shade, in a pattern to your preference.

o   Spritz with fixing spray.

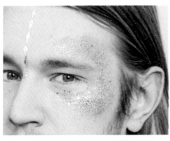
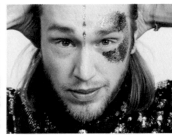
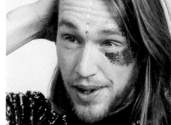
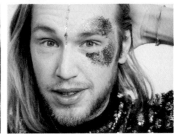
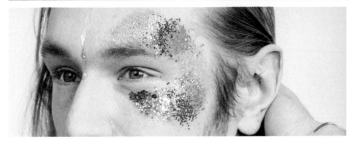

'EVERYBODY LOVES
THINGS THAT SPARKLE.'

Philip Treacy

15

FRECKLES WITH SPARKLY SPECKLES

15
FRECKLES WITH SPARKLY SPECKLES

This take on freckles is nothing short of fabulous. How far you want to take it will depend on whether you choose to precisely apply a few individual sequins or instead dust many more over your nose and beyond.

What you need:

Fine-particle cosmetic glitter or individual sequins

Fixing spray

Make-up brush

o Once your usual make-up look is complete, apply glitter to the end of the make-up brush and gently dust it across cheeks. For this, we'd suggest keeping it scant for a cleaner, gentler take.

✕ Spritz with fixing spray.

✕

'BEING A STAR JUST MEANS THAT YOU FIND YOUR OWN SPECIAL PLACE, AND THAT YOU SHINE WHERE YOU ARE.'

Dolly Parton

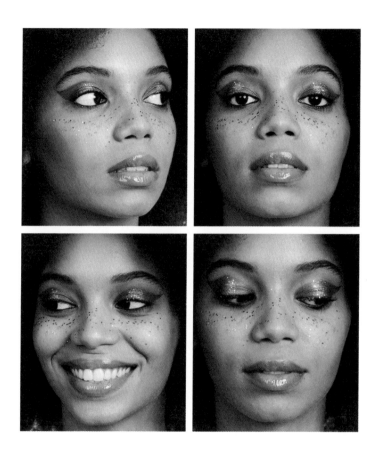

16

THE GLITTER GRADE

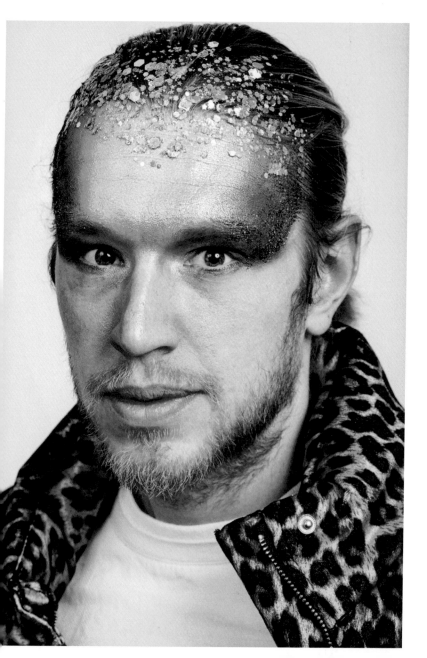

16
THE GLITTER GRADE

This look takes a fabulous eye effect to the extreme. Evolving way past the brow bones and into the hairline, this is a look that takes it to the next level. Don't think you need to team it with a dramatic eye; a simple slick of black mascara with the sequins can make for an effective evolution of the usual glitter beauty style.

What you need:

Hairspray

Make-up glue

Gems

Cosmetic glitter

Cosmetic sequins

Glitter hairspray

Comb

- o Using the comb and hairspray, slick back your hair from the parting. Here is when you would begin to create the desired make-up look, whether that's a bold superhero style or more painterly pastels.

- ✂ Apply the gems with the glue on the skin (not working close to the eyes), and also in the hair.

- . Fix the hair section with more hairspray.

- o Once the gems are securely attached, spray over the glitter hairspray. Apply glue and sprinkle more glitter, sequins and sparkle on top.

- o Finish with more hairspray to hold everything in place.

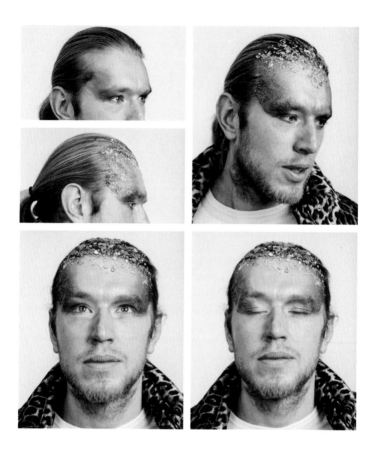

17

SHAPE IT OUT

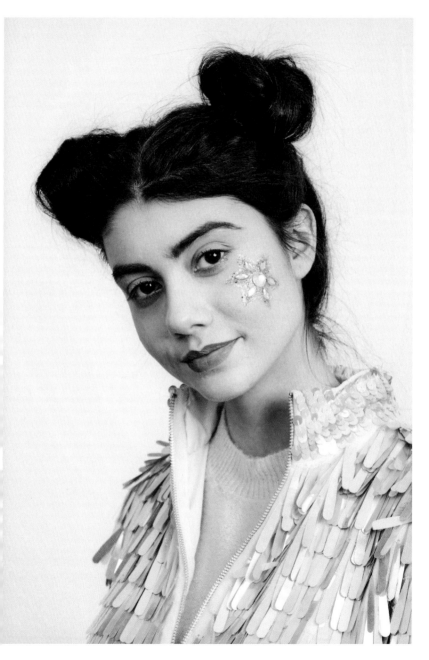

17
SHAPE IT OUT

Here's where glitter gets occasion-appropriate and suitably seasonable. These tips will enable you to create whichever shape feels right for you, right now. A tribute to David Bowie's iconic lightning bolt might fit a festival, or perhaps it's Valentine's Day and you want the look of love? Whatever it might be, this effective style, once mastered, is bound to be the envy of all your pals.

What you need:

Eyeliner	Cosmetic glitter
Face paints or eyeshadows, depending on the desired effect	Cosmetic sequins or gems (optional)
	Fixing spray
Make-up glue	Brushes

o On clean skin, mark out your shape with the eyeliner. This could be on a cheek, or over your eyes or lips for a more striking look. Pulling skin taught will help you get a more precise line.

✕ Begin to colour in-between the lines with the face paint or eyeshadow.

. Once dry, apply glue to all, or areas, of the shape, before quickly adding glitter.

o Once that has set, use extra glue to apply gems or sequins, if required.

-¦- Spritz with fixing spray to finish the look.

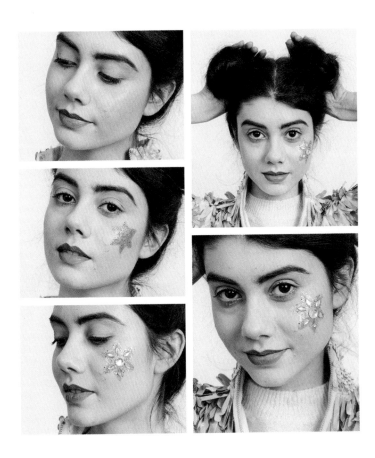

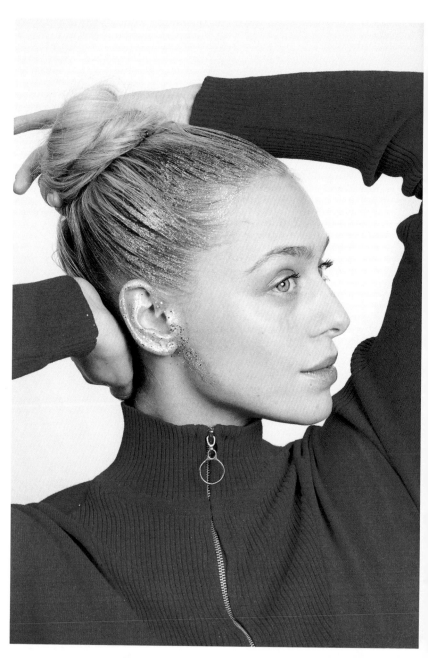

18

GLITTER GLOWING EARS

18
GLITTER GLOWING EARS

Trust us on this one. It's become a catwalk favourite over the last few years, and if you're already one who loves a lot of ear candy, this will take it one step – okay, maybe a few more – further.

What you need:

Make-up glue

Cosmetic glitter

Fixing spray

Brush

Cotton pad

o Following the natural curve of your ear, apply the glue where and how much you want it.

✕ Before the glue dries, apply the glitter.

. Wipe away any excess glitter with the cotton pad, before spritzing with a fixing spray.

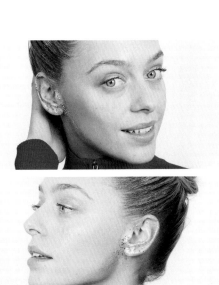

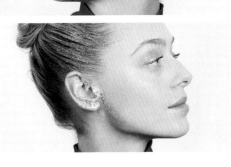

'NOTHING CAN DIM THE LIGHT
THAT SHINES FROM WITHIN.'

Maya Angelou

19
GLITTER UNDER EYE

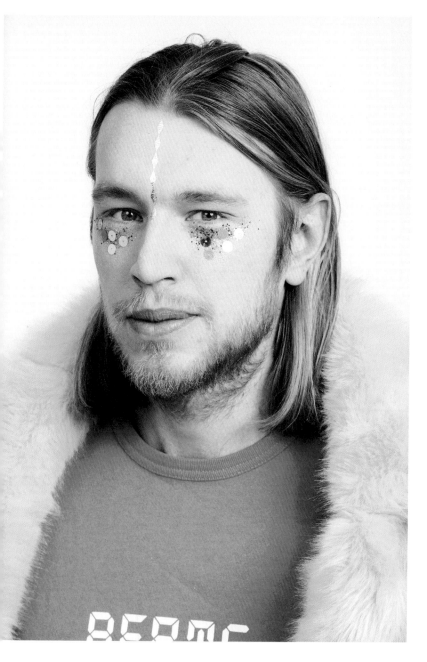

19
GLITTER UNDER EYE

Up all night with nothing
to shine about? No worries.
Cover dark circles with glitter
for a whole new talking point
that can quickly lead to another
nocturnal adventure …

What you need:

Make-up glue

Cosmetic glitter and/or sequins

o Using your fingertips, apply
the glue under the eye, being
watchful of the waterline.

-¦- Using clean, dry fingertips,
gently dab the glitter as
intensely or as sparsely as
you wish, adding sequins
over the top with a little
more glue if you like.

'YOU CAN'T JUST
SIT THERE AND WAIT
FOR PEOPLE TO GIVE
YOU THAT GOLDEN
DREAM. YOU'VE GOT
TO GET OUT THERE
AND MAKE IT HAPPEN
FOR YOURSELF.'

-¦- **Diana Ross**

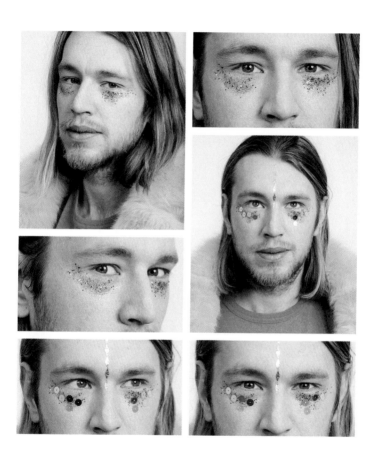

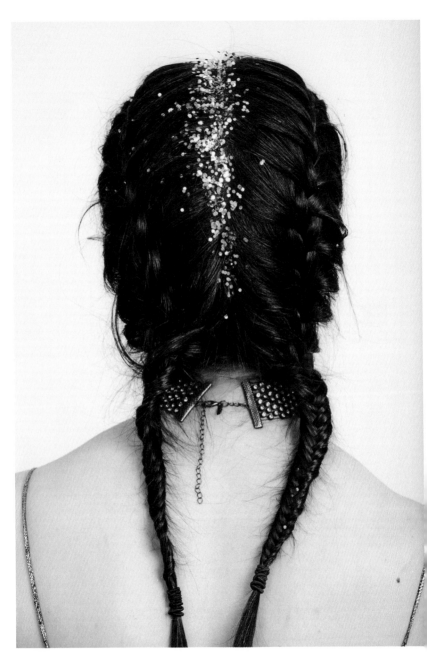

20

GORGEOUS
GLITTER ROOTS

20
GORGEOUS GLITTER ROOTS

Are you really having a good time if you've not got glitter in your hair? No look feels more dancefloor ready than glitter roots. Easy to do yourself, but more fun to do for friends; it's you, but on a really fabulous hair day.

What you need:

Spray-in hair colour (optional)

Hairspray

Glitter or confetti

Comb

o Start by perfecting your parting with the thin end of the comb – you'll find that day-old hair is best for this style.

✕ With the parting in place, get creative by spraying the optional colour along the hairline. Concentrate on the parting and then comb the shade through the roots.

. Next, liberally apply hairspray. This will keep both the colour and the glitter in place, so don't be afraid to be generous, but not overzealous.

o Sprinkle glitter along the parting and place larger sequins strategically across.

⌐⌐ Secure with more hairspray.

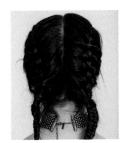
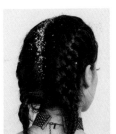
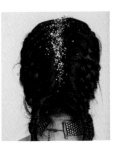
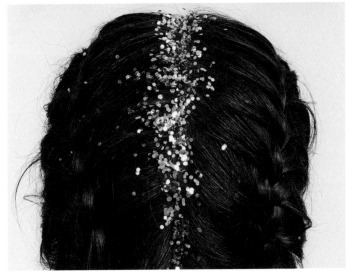

21

BEDAZZLED BRAIDS

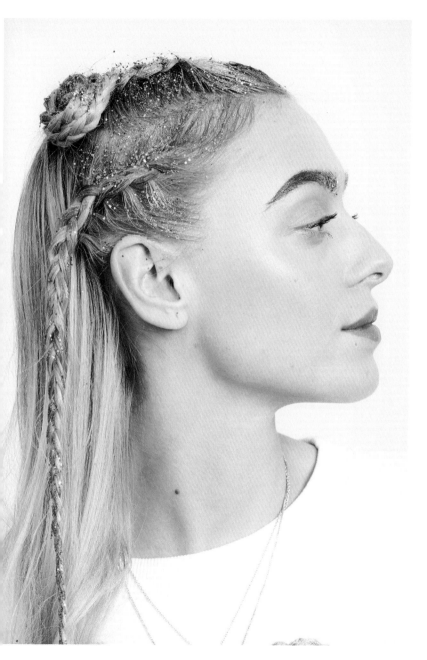

21
BEDAZZLED BRAIDS

Whether you're a pro at braiding or slowly getting to grips with a pair of French plaits, an explosion of sparkle will take your twists to the next level. You want the whole lengths to be sparkling evenly, so another pair of hands will be useful, unless you have eyes in the back of your head …

What you need:

Hair bobbles

Glitter hair gel

Hairspray

Loose glitter

Paintbrush

Comb

o Once you've chosen your braided style, fasten with colourful bobbles for a kaleidoscopic finish.

✕ Working from the top of the plaits, start by painting on the glitter gel, focusing on the centre and working outwards.

. Once all the lengths are coated, fix with hairspray and, when it's setting, sprinkle over the loose glitter powder.

o Finish with an extra coat of hairspray.

'YOU KNOW YOU'RE LIVING RIGHT WHEN YOU WAKE UP, BRUSH YOUR HAIR – AND CONFETTI FALLS OUT.'

Katy Perry

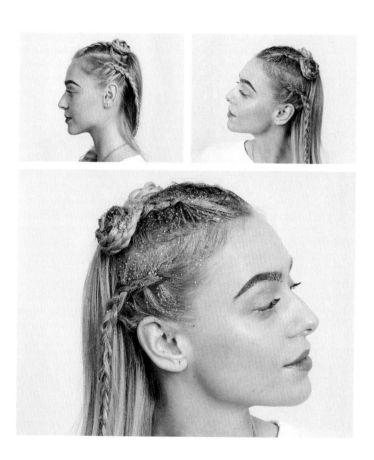

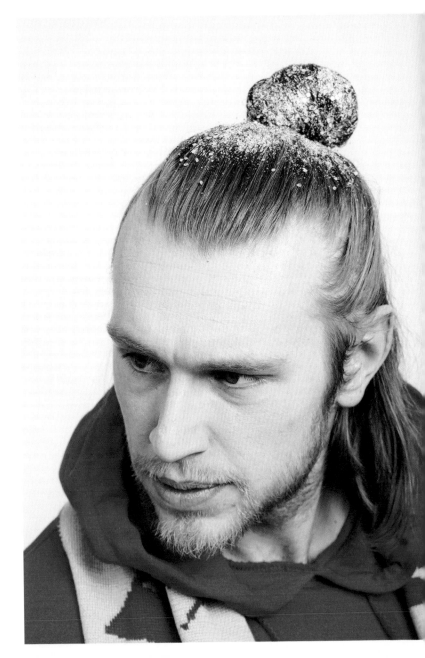

22

GLITTER BUN

22
GLITTER BUN

Everything is better dipped in a little something sparkly. The same applies to the universally loved hair bun. Man buns might be over, but a glitter man bun – now that's something we can work with.

What you need:

Hairspray

Cosmetic glitter

Hair bobbles

Hairbrush

○ Work the hair into a perfect bun before teasing at it with the brush for a more laidback appearance.

✕ Spray the hairspray liberally over the bun.

. Working quickly, shake the glitter over the bun, covering it entirely, and then working it out through the roots.

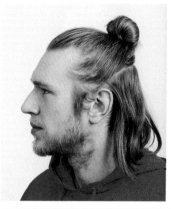
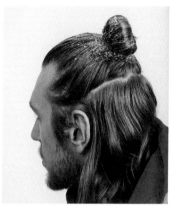
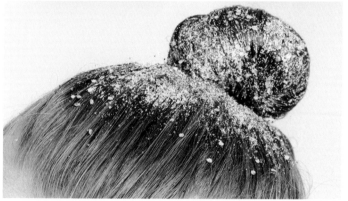

23

STENCIL OUT THE SHINE

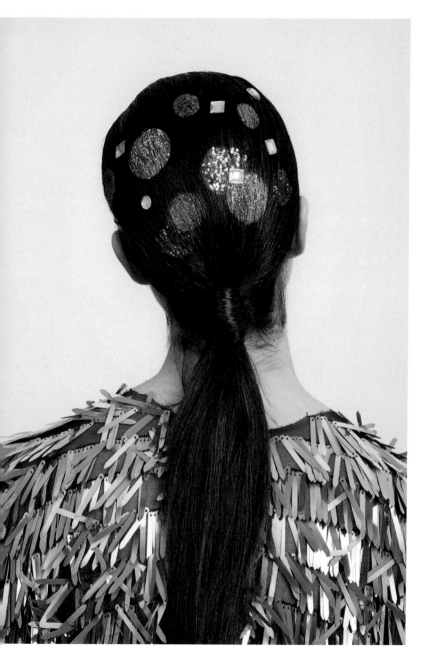

23
STENCIL OUT THE SHINE

Making your own hair stencils will make this look all the more bespoke, but don't disregard ones you can pick up in a craft shop. Change up shapes, sizes and colours for a unique, one-night-only look.

What you need:

Colour hairspray in various shades

Glitter hairspray

Hairspray

Make-up glue

Gems

Stencils

Comb

o Smooth the hair as much as possible and place the stencil over a section. Spray the colour spray over the stencil quickly but neatly.

✕ Next, slightly move the stencil to one side for an alternative pattern and then spray the glitter hairspray through the stencil.

. Finish with a coat of normal hairspray and wait for it all to dry before moving the hair too much. Finish with gems attached here and there with a little glue.

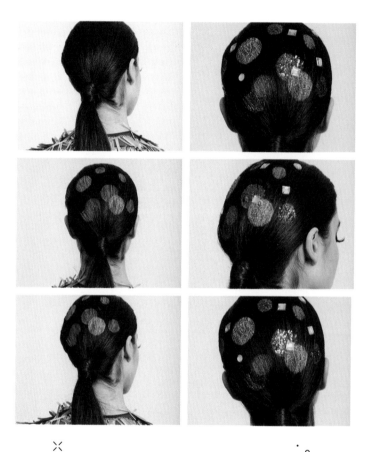

'I HAVE NEVER HATED A MAN ENOUGH
TO GIVE HIM DIAMONDS BACK.'

Zsa Zsa Gabor

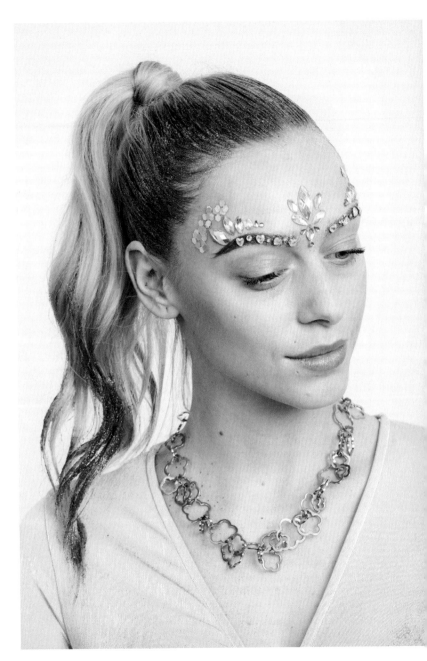

24

THE MERMAID TAIL

24
THE
MERMAID TAIL

Take the magic of sparkle and shimmer under the sea. This style splashes out of Ariel's look book and works best when worn in coral-reef purples or rock-pool blues. Finish with a statement hair bobble or well-tied ribbon for a sweet addition.

What you need:

Hair gel

Cosmetic glitter

Hairspray

Brush

Hair bobbles

o Fasten hair in a ponytail and comb through the length to ensure that it's knot-free.

✕ From about two thirds of the ponytail length down, apply the hair gel to the ends.

. Before the gel sets, apply the loose glitter to the ends, focusing on it being denser at the bottom for a dipped-in effect.

o Fix with hairspray and leave to dry before getting dressed.

TOP TIP:
For the ultimate mermaid moment, start the look once you've already created glitter roots.

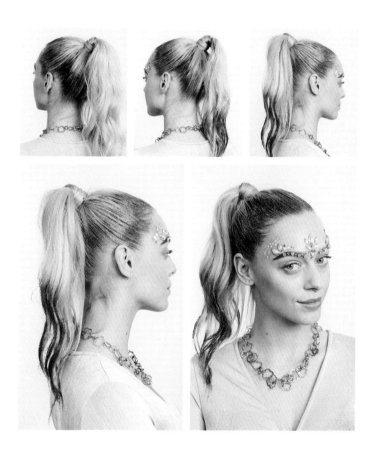

25

THE GLITTER-GLOW BEARD

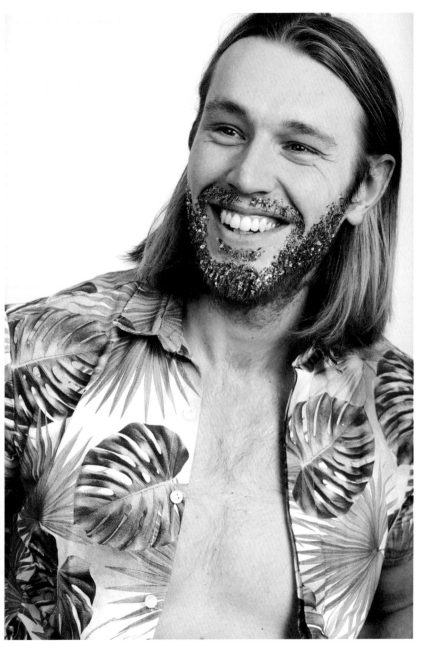

25
THE GLITTER-GLOW BEARD

Granted, you've done the hard work already and grown an impressive face of fuzz, but this look is simpler than one, two, three. In two steps you'll take your beard from bland to bling. Those wanting to up the ante further should think about adding in some earrings that double up nicely as ornaments, or those with shorter facial hair could use an eyeshadow to intensify the base colour.

What you need:

Beard oil

Cosmetic glitter

Spoon

o Apply the beard oil liberally all over your facial hair. The beard oil acts as glue here, so you need to provide enough for the glitter to really stick to.

✂ Fill the spoon with glitter and then shake it all over the beard until it is filled with sparkles. Voila.

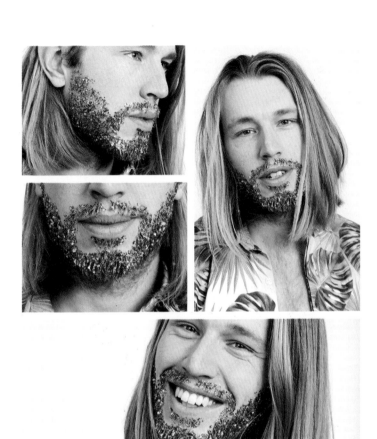

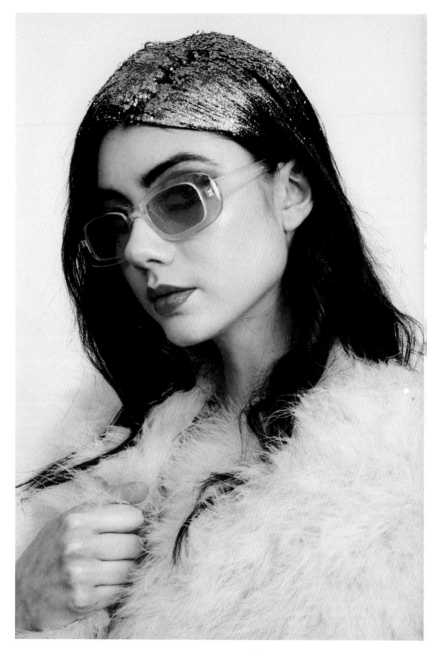

26

GLITTER PARTING

26
GLITTER PARTING

Give the allusion that you're so, so fabulous that glitter literally grows from your roots by turning your parting into your very own blank canvas. Stay away from darker shades and embrace vibrant colours or a pastel palette.

What you need:

Spray-in hair colour

Hairspray

Cosmetic glitter or confetti

Sequins

Tweezers

Comb

o Start by perfecting your parting with the thin end of the comb – you'll find that day-old hair is best for this style.

✕ Spray the colour along the hairline, concentrating on the parting and then combing the shade through the roots.

. Next, liberally hairspray the colour. This will also keep the glitter in place so don't be afraid to be generous.

o Sprinkle a fine glitter along the parting and use the tweezers to place sequins across it. Secure with more hairspray.

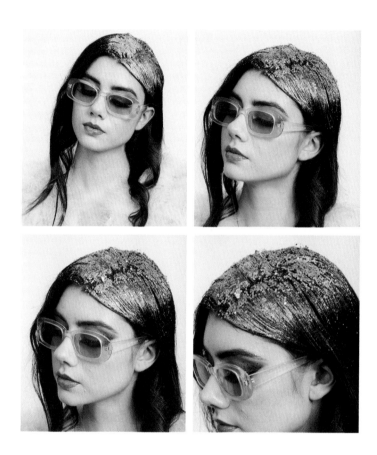

27

MESMERISING
METALLIC MANICURE

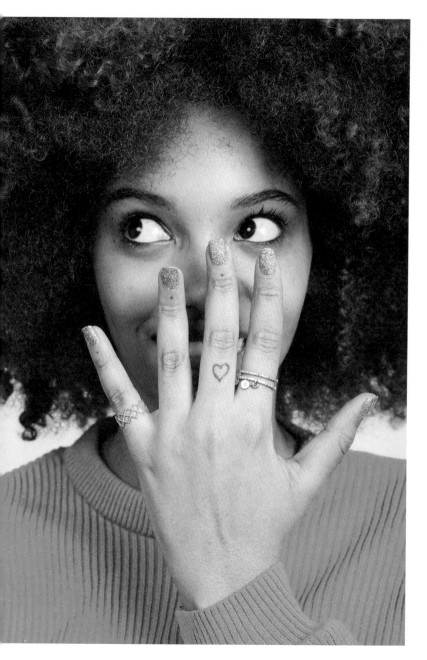

27
MESMERISING METALLIC MANICURE

The one to wear every day. Here, we show you how to master the technique for a perfect glitter-tastic manicure but interpret it as you see fit. Mix colours and shades, glitters and textures, as well as which fingers get the glow for a unique take that will never look the same twice.

What you need:

Coloured nail varnish

Glitter nail varnish

Top coat

Nail-varnish remover

Cotton bud

o Once nails are filed to the desired shape, apply two coats of the colour shade to form a base coat.

✕ When touch-dry, apply the glitter nail varnish. Use shorter strokes for best glitter coverage.

. Finish with a top coat and neaten by removing any excess with nail-varnish remover around the cuticles.

TOP TIP:
For fuller, total glitter coverage, look to YouTuber Kelli Marissa's revolutionising technique: instead of applying the glitter directly to the nail, apply it first to a cosmetic sponge. Trust us, it works!

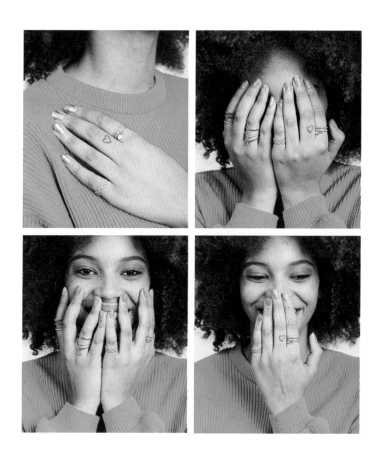

28

FABULOUS FINGERTIPS

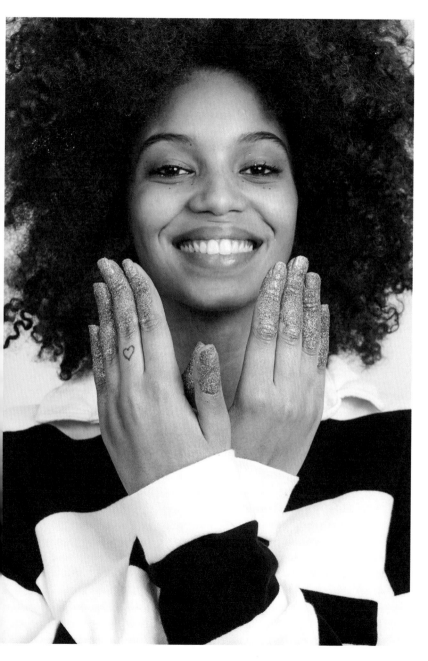

28
FABULOUS FINGERTIPS

If glitter nails just aren't quite satisfying your need for shimmer, then this next step surely will. There's no hiding that this one gets things a little messy, but nothing worth doing has ever been easy now, has it?

What you need:

Make-up glue

Cosmetic glitter

Teaspoon

o Once you've created your glitter nails and they're fully dry (not just touch-dry), apply a thin layer of make-up glue to the tops of your fingertips, all the way to your knuckles. (For neatness, it's best to start by decorating your dominant hand with the glitter.)

. Scoop a teaspoon of glitter and sprinkle it over the fingers so that it catches in the glue.

o For longevity, once dry, don't get wet or agitate the decoration.

TOP TIP:
Use body tape to make
defined edges.

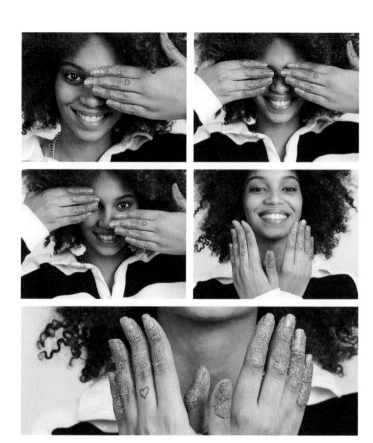

'I'M JUST TRYING TO CHANGE THE
WORLD, ONE SEQUIN AT A TIME.'

Lady Gaga

29

THE GLITTER CAPE

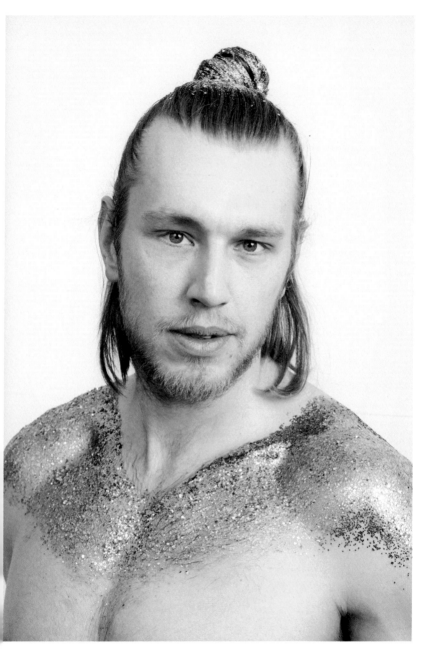

29
THE GLITTER CAPE

Brave the chill and take on the challenge of switching out your actual clothing for a colour explosion of sparkle. Get your pals on board, lay down plenty of protective sheets, and get ready to turn more heads than ever before.

What you need:

Make-up glue

Gems or crystals (optional)

Cosmetic glitter

Fixing spray

Paintbrush

Body tape (optional)

○ If using, start by using the body tape to mark out the shape.

✕ Next, place any gems or crystals strategically to complement your chosen design. Secure with glue.

. Working quickly, apply the glue and then add the glitter with the paintbrush. Use a dabbing motion for a more successful, even application.

╶┼╴ Finish with a spritz of finishing spray.

TOP TIP:
Set out markers with body tape, which can then be removed, for a defined, clear line that makes for a realistic top effect!

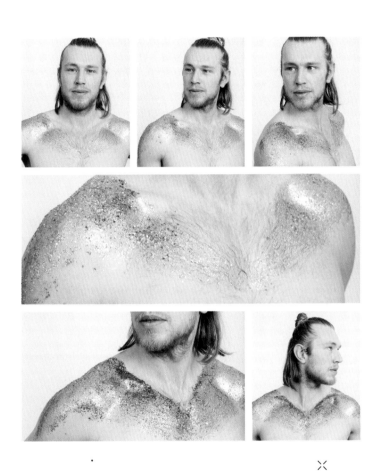

'WE ARE ALL OF US STARS, AND
WE DESERVE TO TWINKLE.'

Marilyn Monroe

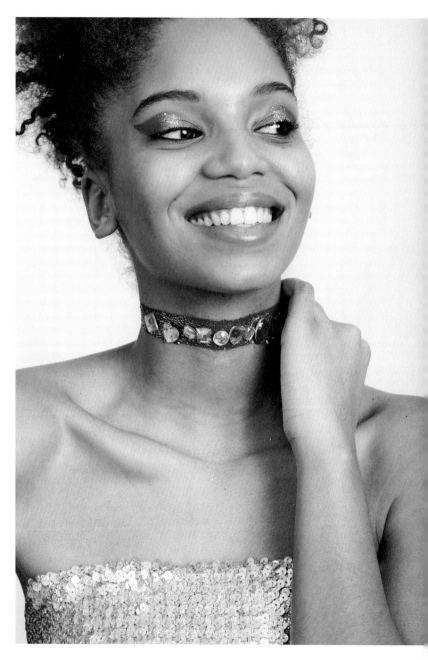

30

SECOND-SKIN
SPARKLE CHOKER

30
SECOND-SKIN SPARKLE CHOKER

Who can resist the nineties' favourite necklace? The perfect accessory to add some retro realness to any look. This will soon become a fast favourite that you can take from festival to disco and, who knows, maybe you'll also dare to wear for day?

What you need:

Body paint

Make-up glue

Cosmetic glitter

Rhinestones

Fixing spray

Two paintbrushes

o Around the middle of your neck, draw a 3cm solid line with the body paint. If you have short hair or intend on wearing it up, ask a friend to help you go all the way around.

✕ Once the paint has dried, apply the glue over the painted line. Then carefully add the glitter, in shades of your choice, over it.

. When the glitter is set, use glue to apply the rhinestones on top of the painted choker.

o Spritz with fixing spray to complete the look.

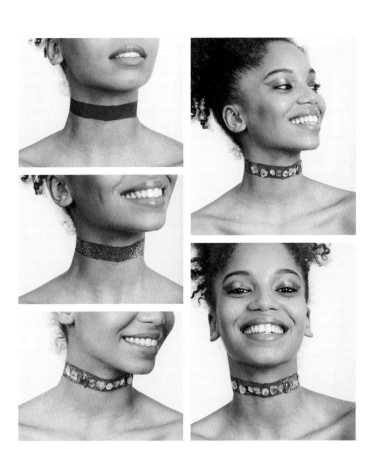

BLINGSTAGRAM

@AADAM_SHEIKH This student is the fashion industry's new favourite follow.

@PATMCGRATHREAL British *Vogue* beauty editor-at-large Pat has amassed seven figure followers.

@S_STELLER_ Glitter lips is a great place to start and Sarah's account has all the inspiration you need.

@WINTERVEA If eyes are your thing, then vegan MUA Victoria is your must-follow. All the products are #crueltyfree.

@GLISTEN_COSMETICS Selling a range of cruelty-free glitters and gels from their online shop, Glisten Cosmetics are experts in the field.

@HEATHERLINESMUA Whether it's a festival or an all-night party look, you'll find it on Heather's eclectic feed.

@NAOKOSCINTU Naoko's feed is a real-life demonstration of the busy life of an in-demand MUA with a considered and curated approach.

@LYNSEYALEXANDER A mastermind of make-up, Lynsey is the brains behind Topshop's most ingenious beauty moments.

@GLITTERONMYTONGUE Sparkle is taken from a festival favourite and repositioned as an art material to provoke and invoke humour.

@SEQUINDESIGNS Embellishing fishnets and decorating pantyhose, these designs are the perfect fuss-free way to liven up an outfit.

1 3 5 7 9 10 8 6 4 2

Pop Press, an imprint of Ebury Publishing,
20 Vauxhall Bridge Road,
London SW1V 2SA

Pop Press is part of the Penguin Random House group of companies whose addresses can be found at global.penguinrandomhouse.com

Penguin
Random House
UK

Text by Naomi Pike © Pop Press 2018

Photography © Ellis Parrinder

Naomi Pike has asserted her right to be identified as the author of this Work in accordance with the Copyright, Designs and Patents Act 1988

Make-up by Lauren Kay
Styling by Jamie Jarvis
Design by Emily Voller
Project editing by whitefox

Clothes from ASOS, Isolated Heroes, Jakke, Fiorucci, Rokit, Monki, Topman, Topshop, Weekday

Modelled by Kora, Miles, Mia and Athena at BMA Models

First published in the United Kingdom by Pop Press in 2018

www.penguin.co.uk

A CIP catalogue record for this book is available from the British Library

ISBN 9781785039379

Colour origination by BORN
Printed and bound in China
by Toppan Leefung

Penguin Random House is committed to a sustainable future for our business, our readers and our planet. This book is made from Forest Stewardship Council® certified paper.